Vibrant Health & Sexual Life Through 140 and Beyond With His Spirit

by

Jay B. Kuennen,

M.D. in Alt. Med., MDH in Homeopathy, MPA, MSW

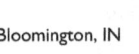

Bloomington, IN

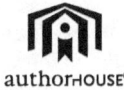

authorHOUSE®

Milton Keynes, UK

AuthorHouse™
1663 Liberty Drive, Suite 200
Bloomington, IN 47403
www.authorhouse.com
Phone: 1-800-839-8640

AuthorHouse™ UK Ltd.
500 Avebury Boulevard
Central Milton Keynes, MK9 2BE
www.authorhouse.co.uk
Phone: 08001974150

First published by AuthorHouse 2/22/2007

ISBN: 978-1-4259-8342-0 (sc)

Printed in the United States of America
Bloomington, Indiana

This book is printed on acid-free paper.

This book is not intended to replace the services of a physician, nor is it meant to encourage diagnosis and treatment of illness, diseases, or other medical problems by the nonprofessional. Any application of the recommendations set forth in the following pages are at the reader's discretion and sole risk. If you are under a physician's care for any condition, he or she can advise you whether the program described in this book is suitable for you.

CONTENTS

FOREWORD

So what? This writing in chapter 1 is a pathway designed for us to follow should we want a mental, physical, and spiritual way of being at our top performance and health. We all know we are and will be challenged in ever increasing ways with our environmental shifts. Virus strains, epidemics, and other catastrophic events ... 9/11, Katrina, and the recent past tsunami, impact our survival chances. With sensitivity to these phenomena we will want to be more self-actualized with Hope.

Is it important to look at the mind, body, and spirit condition to fulfill our longevity potentials? Chapter 2 helps us know how Positive Mental Attitude with exercise, nutritional balance through Science, and a clear sense of ones own vital energy and longevity brings outcomes. Knowledge is a key and taking charge is essential. Hope is always an integral part of this process. Desired is that this chapter opens the sense of hope in a stronger way!

In western society we get distracted at times. Staying focused is a central theme in chapter 3. Eat, sleep, take vitamins, minerals, herbs, healthy foods, super foods, do 10,000 steps a day – briskly, and pray or meditate daily – one to three hours a day. Have fun and challenge yourself in learning how to double your life span with good health. Be challenged to chase your dreams through 140 years or more.

Do we have the right to self-treat or should the courts decide treatment for us? This is perhaps central to our health and longevity as brought out in chapter 4. In which order should we consider our health care needs. If we first choose invasive chemicals that can over power and block curative medicines, then what can be done? How can we stand up to the traditionalist doctors and the weight of their medical association? We must understand it can be critically important to choose curative versus invasive and or symptom management medicines. Why this is important is found in chapter 4.

Chapter 5 encourages us to reach our full potential NOW and have empowered good health to 140 and beyond. Will it be natural, alternative medical solutions for preventive and healthful living or allopathic medicine that can block choices for cure?

PREFACE

The importance of this book is that it is a guide to healthy living, avoiding illnesses, and Lord forbid, having a major health problem, then, knowing which kind of health care professional to first turn for information and help. The author brings knowledge and concepts together from others who represent separate and yet similar thinking. The list of references cited bring about confidence we can and ought to live much longer lives in good health. To date it is rare to read a book that gives the combined health information with a method to decide what medical doctoring to turn to first. In addition the author guides decisions we make based on knowing ourselves best and then a way to take care of ourselves first. Is this a basic right or will the traditional doctors through the courts take that away from the individual? Will we continue to be able to go down to a store and buy an aspirin or an herb or will we have to go to a traditional doctor for a prescription, first?

ACKNOWLEDGEMENTS

To my grandparents, parents, children, grandchildren, a very special and significant lady – Aida, and special friends who have persisted with me having and maintaining good habits. There are many others who I think of with special affections, my brothers, sisters, their spouses, their children, my aunts and uncles, cousins, and friends. I have a special thanks to Sir Dr. Malik A. Kaiyoom Awan who was my proctor for several years. Also, I thank my friends with whom I have worked with these past many years and am now living in early retirement. I give thanks to God as his steward in all I do. Each give me the fortitude and faith to continue my research and care of others.

INTRODUCTION

Countless books and sources of information are at our fingertips in the quest to reduce our risk of illness, prolong our life span, look younger, have better sex or plainly just perform our daily routines with more than enough energy to last the day. That has been my journey until I came to know Dr. Jay with his approach to maintain vibrant health through nutritional and cell renewal.

In his small book, Dr. Jay has dedicated years of study and experience to assemble a direct approach to enhance our body's performance and learn realistically how to add many years to our lives naturally and without too much confusion. As you read his book you must understand that you, and you alone are the creator of your own health according to His Will. We have the power to control and make the necessary steps with determination and care to heal, enhance, beautify and strengthen our bodies. Dr.

Jay's vast knowledge of preventive medicine and natural healing has convinced me that the best way to stay away from hospitals or orthodox doctors is to empower yourself with knowledge of nature's own remedies and apply this knowledge.

It doesn't matter if you are a young person in your twenties or a middle age person. It doesn't matter if you are wealthy or not; have a good doctor or good genes; it doesn't matter what kind of life style you have had prior to reading his book. Prepare your mind, body and spirit to live healthier and longer, as our thoughts and convictions also have tremendous effect in how we approach the multitude of choices and circumstances that we face every day.

Having experienced some health issues in my thirties, I wanted to find out how I could limit or eliminate the risks of serious illness. I don't like pain, needles, and especially I don't like the dreaded feeling of not knowing what the results on a test or X rays will be. So, I have been on the search of knowledge reading all I could from nutrition to spiritual books and all the many aspects of health and well-being. Dr. Jay introduced me to the idea of *maintaining a well-functioning immune system in a natural way.* After following his advice for almost two years and noticing the benefits of his method, I've came to the conclusion that no one is able to know how many years one will live, but we can definitely help and provide our bodies with the elements to sustain a strong, healthy body through many years of quality life, as Doctor Jay asserts: to as much as 140 years or more!

CHAPTER 1

The Need

Are you ready for quality life through 140? We are in a time of high need to be ready. There are continuous alerts regarding terrorist threats, threats of new virus strains: SAR's to news reports of scientists who are developing new stains of virus to sell to governments that can invade whole communities quietly and leave no trace, threats of epidemics as bird flu, hepatitis and aids. So, how ready can we individually become?

Since 9/11, the Trade Center disaster we have been experiencing an alarming need to be ready for any kind of event including biological warfare. We are getting many pieces of information daily in the news and sometimes several times each day these matters can reach our attention through the news. Never before have we been in a heads-up ball game in life. We each need for our physical survival and our spiritual survival to be in top shape physically, mentally, and spiritually. We need to be social advocates to each other and be involved in our communities to be more fit and prepared to deal with such concerns.

New forms of dangers present themselves sometimes from unknown sources as in Specific Absorption Rate SAR's, i.e. through cellular phones. Scientists are learning more about this one. Deadly virus as eboli, bird flu, encephalitis, aids, cancer, and various cardiac diseases are threatening our lives. We are informed by news medias' that scientists are creating new dangerous strains for purchase! Scary as this is, how do we preserve, prevent, and survive those and other health challenges today? We know our leadership persons can do a great deal, for example, in the search for high criminals and in the out come with the Iraqi 21 day war. Many of our religious leaders agree we are in the period of the "end millennium". This agreement seems to be based upon many signs of this era, the scriptural interpretations tempered with some scientific knowledge. Are we facing an apocalypse or will humankind, as amazing as we are, find non-violent and healthful solutions?

What is it in one person who remains healthy and another who gets sick when exposed to the same virus? Through our senses, experience, and developed knowledge we get our understanding or maybe some clues. Our individual sciences and combined sciences yield more clues. Steven Cherniske in The Metabolic

Plan identifies our endocrine system having a great deal to do with health and living longer. Miracles and other unexplained phenomena through faith healing can yield more clues. Can we learn to trust our senses, our experiences, and our knowledge as a way to be prepared? What are our inalienable rights as we continue to evolve in prevention of illnesses and providing health care services? Our Allopathic doctors want and will insist on our signing a medical release of liability should we not take their advice and/or prescribed medication. We as persons and individuals in society may be abdicating the responsibilities to ourselves when we only rely on one legitimate form of health care. Our current prevailing form of western medicine is allopathic and organized through the American Medical Association and the health care system. In some of our united states this is the only legitimate licensable form of medicine. Yet through the recognized world there is at least two other major medical forms, Homeopathic medicine and Ayurvedic medicine. There are other practiced forms of health care, for example, naturopathy and herbal remedies. Do we as individuals rely too much on our traditional doctors of medicine, this may be truer in the United States. You may have many more such questions. For example, do we, you and I, have an inalienable right to not just know these various medical specialties, but also treat ourselves?

Of course, this idea of self-treatment is in light of when it is prudent and possible.

Sometimes the idea of self-treatment won't work: especially if one is pulled from an auto wreck with broken bones!

Do our present farming techniques give us all we need for our mineral and vitamin intake? Over time it is asserted our soils in the United States have become depleted of many minerals, some assert since the 1930's. Our soils do not contain the rich variety of minerals even with fertilizers that add back into the soil. Some of our farmers refuse to use certain fertilizers because they may have contaminants as a way of spreading these over large open areas to increase the half-life of the contaminants. So, how can we possibly be getting these necessary minerals in our foods? We can't. Our food sources are not as enriched as they were, even in our grandparent's days. Yet, we are facing phenomena in our society that creates stress in much greater proportions. Is it little wonder we see people stressing out, breaking down with social and mental illnesses. Is it little wonder we can't fight off viruses and other maladies in our time? If our body is not getting what it needs, how can we expect our brains to work well and our minds to be at our peak performance. How can we keep our thinking and spiritual welfare at full readiness? For many of us we may need our minds, bodies, and spirits revived up and empowered for the many challenges ahead.

One of this countries outspoken Doctor's is Doctor Weil. He advocates alternative health and has shared a story of a gentleman who shared it with him. It has to do with a man who describes a healthy river. Over time this river became polluted such that it could not support life. Chemicals from factories, sewage, etc. changed it from a healthy river to a dead river. Dr Weil goes on to say we can and do revive rivers! Reducing and eliminating pollutants in rivers can revive rivers - just as we can renew our body systems.

The "Family Medical Guide" relates there are six basic rules for healthy living: 1) If you smoke, quit. This is a strong factor in coronary heart disease and in cancers of the lung, mouth, esophagus, throat, bladder, and cervix. It also accelerates aging of the skin, bones, and lungs. 2) Don't drink alcohol but in moderation. Drink none if you are pregnant or operate machinery. If you have a problem get help through your doctor. While drugs, street drugs, or misuse of drugs are off limits. 3) Find some exercise you enjoy. Recommended is swimming or walking at least 30 minutes each time - daily or four to six times a week. (It is good to set a goal of up to 10,000 steps each time or four to six times a week. 10,000 steps is up to 5 miles). You can divide this into smaller segments (but it is recommended not to do less than 2500 steps in each segment). 4) Eat a wide variety of natural foods. Include many whole grains, fresh fruit, and fresh vegetables. Use moderation with fatty foods. 5) Keep your body trim. Do not let yourself get overweight. Obesity is linked to many serious disorders as heart disease and diabetes mellitus. If you are overweight, try hard to make permanent changes in your eating habits and life style. And, 6) Have a regular medical check-up. It could be a time for a paradigm shift!

While AMA in the "Family Medical Guide" presented a good basic reference, a health conscious person will go further. To be empowered in good health we each need a broader and deeper perspective. I suggest in this part of our search we enhanced vitamins and minerals up to 100 + or - daily. Additional food supplements can wonderfully enrich our efforts with a little extra reading on herbs. Dr Kirschner in the 1940's and 1950's formulated the "Green Drink". In chapter 3 I reference this wonderful drink and enrich it with bringing more to it as a way to fortify us against invading viruses and maintaining better health. More writers, including myself, believe we each need a strong spiritual centeredness along life's journey. Research reveals that if we lack a spiritual centeredness, we can become susceptible to many illnesses and diseases.

To become empowered in a pro-active health program

we have to talk about enhanced vitamins and minerals that go above the minimum daily requirement. And, when we have known family weaknesses, i.e. cancer, diabetes, etc. certain vitamin and minerals will need to be carefully considered.

Dr Giller, M.D. broke each of the main vitamin and minerals down in his "Medical Makeover". He gives a good way to assess our own requirement. His book dealt with the basic group of vitamin and minerals we all have come to be acquainted with in a "one-a-day". Having said this if we come to know and understand herbs then we can know there are natural sources as well as formulated sources - those that come in tablets, etc. The herbs often go beyond and offer much more. With this discussion is the realization we need to eat good nutritional foods, balanced, in our daily diet. We should eat appropriate portions of three to five meals a day. Dr Kirschner's book informs us and gives us an excellent way to integrate herbs and their value to us nutritionally in his "Green Drink". Thanks to Stephen Cherniske in The Metabolic Plan we can now reason how our endocrine system can also be a catalyst to longevity, his plan shows us a better way, too!

With the turn of this century and the new millennium religious fervor has greatly increased. The vigilance that has come from this period still remains in many faithful minds. There is speculation we are in the end period or end millennium. Many religions and religious leaders acknowledge we could be in this period of time. This presents another reason we want to strengthen our minds with the best nutritional readiness for clarity of mind and spirit to deal with these eventualities. This will be discussed more in my next chapter.

Ever heard of El Nino? What? El Nino is a weather phenomena caused by growth in warm water mass in the Pacific Ocean. This warming effect causes a type of fungus that contaminates shellfish and makes them inedible. Birds are becoming infected. These types of reports are more common in our newspapers and on TV news. Some have speculated this warm body of water will present even worse weather, than in 1997 in California and other parts of the US and world. In the spring of 2003 we have seen many devastating results from tornados. These phenomena will undoubtedly cause reaction to people as well. We have experienced a Tsunami, which has shifted our world ½ degree on our rotating axis. We have experienced some of the worst hurricanes and most numerous tornados. It is my hope you and I with our enhanced immune system will be ready.

On scene is a new flu virus called SARS. In central California we are alerted to mosquitoes that can carry encephalitis and has at different times, this disease seems to be on the increase. Should we be alert, ready, or wait till in contact with and threatened by these diseases?

We need to learn what to eat, how much to eat, and how often to eat for building maximum prevention capacity in our bodies. We need to know if these foods can yield what we need, even from the best foods! If not, then what can we do to get any deficiencies remedied? How can we get a clear idea of a basic readiness for ourselves, each of us being different with potentially different requirements? Next, we have to consciously plan our sleeping habits as part of this balance for better health readiness.

Psychotic episodes occur from sleep deprivation. Sometimes knowing such a basic aid to better sleep is to place our head in a north position and our feet in a south position. Our Native American Indian heritage teaches this as being consistent with our natural electro-magnetic processes and keeps us in harmony with mother earth.

What happens when we are under too much stress? What happens when we do not get enough of the correct sustenance over a lifetime? When do we know we should seek professional help? Is there a way to know from whom we should seek professional medical help? When should we treat ourselves or seek professional medical assistance? If we decide to treat ourselves, is this an inalienable right. With our present age of information and computerization - the Internet, can you and I become well enough informed? Can we get this information and rely on it? Yes, in many cases! However, if we are in an automobile accident, we probably ought to go to a good trauma center.

More and more writers are suggesting we should expect longer life spans. In 1997 Harry Stout from the Annuity Store writes ..."as many as one million baby boomers will live to age 100. ...thanks to advanced medical technology and healthier life styles."

One of my goals in this small book is to enlighten and extend the process of expecting longer life, through teaching and learning to live longer through age 165 and beyond. With technology, the Internet, and the availability of knowledge at our fingertips I believe all peoples will have potential for such longevity. As human beings this is an inalienable right to which we should cleave. Under God and through Him we are obliged to live full healthy lives. We ought to become more self-activated and self-actualized with a long life expectation, yet the traditional view is most of us will live into our seventies or eighties. Allopathic Doctoring in the United States tends to control which medical view prevails. Through our institutional and political practices our health choices are heavily controlled and regulated through managed care providers. As good as this system is, in my opinion it is singularly and dangerously myopic. It excludes open and cooperative practices in naturopathic solutions and in alternative medicine. Alternative medicine practice includes broader solutions and is more proactive toward preserving health and prevention of illnesses. Alternative medicines by their nature are less invasive. Traditional medical schools are only recently beginning to educate these points of view. Traditional Doctoring seems egocentric and self-serving - how many allopathic doctors would refer to an alternative medical doctor? Yet many patients do not even get this choice because of the control and influence of AMA and licensure. Life and death choices are made, many, Lord forbid, die because the regular Doctor will most likely not refer a patient outside their field of medicine. Yet... we should all reach ages 120, 140, and 160!

In 1995 Dr Marcus Laux wrote we should all reach ages of 120 to 130. He wrote that we know through modern medicine and nutrition this is a reality. Personally, I believe we all owe it to ourselves to become determined and pursue our full life potential. In today's society, societies, and nations there should be no professional medical or legal barriers that exclude free choice. Medical choice should be accessible to all who decide their conscience without financial barriers. This book is a short, direct, and made affordable to anyone who wants it. It is a guide to make more reasoned choices for medical care.

It is hoped everyone will become more empowered with knowledge made available. This brief introduction, hopefully, will set a stage, a sort of "heads up", a "reviving-up" through individual strength and self-empowerment. Let us all expect to live a minimum of 130 to 165 and in good health that is to live free of wheel chairs and living in our own homes, not in nursing homes! Should these matters catch the attention of a younger person, all the better. Anyone who is twenty, even younger for example, needs to start now. This applies to each of us, at any age. If you have already begun this process great! This can be a new challenge, a new paradigm, or a new point of view!

CHAPTER 2:

What Do You Need?

Knowledge: Mind, Body, and Spirit = Healthful Empowered Living

It is my hope and belief those who get this book will have common sense abilities that will provide ways to know how to achieve a quality life well beyond 120 years of age. With some briefness this chapter will be a short "how to" chapter.

First and foremost, I recommend a growing expanding spiritual relationship to God. Through this kind of commitment each person can achieve extra-rational strength with all one can do. This will give a focus and strength of purpose in life. In working in health care services for over 30 years I have become aware of a profound sense of a lack of purpose in many persons lives. Through these years I have worked with many who have emotional difficulties. Often many have little awareness they have a *purpose* in life. Some are single, married, married with children, single with children, and some live with significant person(s) in their lives. Often many have expressed feelings of being lost or lacking a sense of direction. It is my belief a strong sense of purpose is paramount to longevity. Most people now know many medical scientists are stating we should live to over 100 years of age. Many biologists know we are genetically encoded to live to over 400 years. The closest evidence of this is the reported life of a man who is reputed to have lived 256 years. He died around 1930! And, there are the references in the Old Testament. Presently five cultural groups in our world are people reported to live to 120 - 140 years of age as frequent occurrences! Not since the Old Testament have there been references to such life spans! So, why don't we strive for such life? When asked, many remark: I don't think I want to live that long!

The second greatest attribute we each need to have is good mental health. We need to know how to nourish our minds, not just our brains. In addition to good nutritional balance we must pursue good mental activity, like a great gymnast who works out every day to keep athletic perfection. One hour to three hours a day ought to be a goal. Doing things like puzzles, word games, reading books, spiritual books, playing checkers, chess, etc. It could be any one or more other enjoyable and worthy pursuits of ones choosing.

Third, physical health is a must even if we are in a wheel chair. There are many experts with any one or more recommended programs for most all circumstances. The most universal exercise is walking or swimming for one half an hour one or more times a day. Reaching one to five miles a day at a speed of 3-5 mph or its equivalent is desired. Remember, it is important to commit to a plan that is enjoyable and stick to it. Changing your exercise may be refreshing from time to time, as long as it is enhancing your program. Some strenuous exercise is encouraged – if you need to, check with your doctor first.

The fourth dimension is committing to a long life, baring unforeseen or accidental circumstances. If you are first thinking about or have been thinking about it this book should be encouraging. If you have not yet made this decision then, the challenge is to do so at this very moment. I have confidence God will give His blessing! Develop and/or use your own positive mental attitude (PMA) when making this decision. Expect this to come about in your own life, expect it to happen too, own this expectation! Owning this expectation I believe to be part of the secret to longevity.

Traditional medicine often omits this in their approach to health and care for others. Which allopathic Doctor (Traditional Doctor) that you know of has personally spent two hours taking a new case history? Many may spend ten to fifteen minutes. Maintaining good health, prevention of illness, and other remedies often go unattended from not getting adequate histories. Yet many people assume "they" will give correct advice. Taking time to gather a person's medical history including your parents and grandparent's history is not usually considered. A thorough history including your aunts, and uncles can be very important. Perhaps you have unhealthy habits as smoking, drinking alcohol, sweetened drinks - sodas, caffeine beverages including coffee, etc. I hope you realize you need to stop doing these things that are destructive in your body. Realize the orthodox (traditional) Doctor treats illnesses and diseases after the fact. This is their specialty. Keeping ourselves well is our business and we can get good advice from Naturopathic Doctors (N.D.), Alternative Medical Doctors, and other Specialists. It seems an exception when a traditional (allopathic, orthodox) Doctor in western society especially, will engage in prevention advice - maintaining good health through 165.

Our challenge is to survive incredible new and old strains of viruses, illness, and diseases known and not yet known. Our immune system is being attacked and challenged by viruses and diseases as eboli, aids, encephalitis, SARS, and cancer, to name but a few. We, you and I, must stay vigilant! It is imperative. I believe we can learn how to build and keep our immune system functioning at maximum levels. We are all learning more about antioxidants and how they safeguard our health system. We ought to learn and continue to learn everything we can to boost our immune system and our total health! The Metabolic Plan discusses many concepts, so knowledge of our endocrine system and how anabolic metabolism is important. We need to know how DHEA and the 7-keto, a natural metabolite of DHEA, are important to longevity and good health.

We should know what our *vital force* is! Dr. Hahneman is known as the father of Homeopathy, his whole premise of medicine was based on this principle. Briefly, vital force is that energy which maintains life in a person. He maintained this force is unique in every person, each being endowed with his or her own quantity of it. Vitalism is a principle distinct from chemical or physical forces.

Let's "empower" our lives and celebrate each year, doubly so, for each year over 100! There will be more clues in chapter 3!

CHAPTER 3

How to Do It!

Eat, Sleep, take vitamins, minerals, herbs, eat healthy foods, drink super foods, exercise, and pray in The Spirit!

How many of us have committed to the art and science of eating <u>well</u> planned fully balanced meals – super charged? If you are one of the few, do you also realize, these nourishments will still lack adequate nutritional value? What do I mean, you may be thinking? Many experts are now saying our soil lacks nutrients for growing good healthy vegetables, etc. We grow our foods in soil inadequate of the rich ingredients that were there a hundred years ago. These same soils are replete of the nutrition from repeated farm use. Thus, what we eat is just not as rich in nutritions. The foods we grow need to transfer those nutrients to us for our better health and longevity. It is critical to adjust or compensate for this phenomenon. I used to recommend we take a good multiple vitamin and mineral supplement. This supplement should be from a reputable maker and be at a level for an athletic person or for an active person. The amounts of the vitamins and minerals in this formula are higher than in a standard one-a-day type and come closer to meeting our actual needs. Yet, we need more. In The Metabolic Plan we learn of a way to nourish our needs through science and bring super foods for our daily requirements. It is important we come to know and understand those principles discussed. We should also know that supplementing with a *colloidal* mineral formulation that has up to 70 or more trace minerals, negatively charged, is also an important consideration. There are some good manufacturers of these trace minerals. Seven of these trace minerals are reputed to provide another prospect for doubling our life span - to 120 through140 years of age.

It is good to be alert and make adjustments through our lives in addition to the above optimal planning. At times we may be challenged by our genetic weaknesses' and or be challenged by our environment with air and water pollution challenges. The Metabolic Plan has a chapter on organized water; this book is an important reference to have as we seek greater health and longevity.

Basically, we should ensure our daily plan has an ardent *antioxidant* program. We can accomplish much of this through eating of herbs. I suggest we begin by reading about herbs and purchase a few good references on herbs, and update them from time to time. Much is being written about herbs today so take some time and satisfy yourself about the information you are getting. Then, expand your readiness with super foods as discussed in the Metabolic Plan.

How do we protect ourselves from deadly invading viruses? On a day-to-day basis what can we do? A good little book with a wealth of insight is given to us by Dr Kirschner's formula in the 1940's and 1950's. I have added some additional herbs to enrich your reading experience as follows.

The Green Drink - Plus

Dr Kirschner's *Green Drink* with my additions is highlighted below. I recommend you post this on your refrigerator or pantry door, at eye level, as a daily reminder along with your super foods:

> Mint
> Beet Greens
> Radish Leaves
> Spinach Leaves
> Parsley Greens
> Kale Leaves
> Lambs Quarter

Dandelion Greens

Comfrey Leaves, the type approved for consumption, some forms may be injurious to your liver, investigate your selection.

Plus   Alfalfa Greens

Plus   Kelp

Plus   Carrot Top Greens

To put more protein in the drink add these items:

15 Almonds

4 Dates (pitted)

5 Teaspoons of Sunflower Seeds

Now add sufficient pineapple juice (or try a juice of your choice) and place in a liquefier/juicer. Blend till ready, then, store in a refrigerator enough for a day. Drink one to two glasses per day. Make only enough for a day at a time this keeps it fresh and alive for consumption. With the herbs I prefer to purchase them prepared in dry powered form by the pound. If you can raise them in a garden then you can make sandwiches at the same time, a pleasant variation! There is a lot of fun and satisfaction in growing an herb garden! As a reminder place your herbs in air and light tight containers. Always keep in mind the shelf life of these herbs. The proportions of an 8-ounce green drink plus are about 1/4 teaspoon of each herb per glass with pineapple juice or another juice of your choice. Please experiment to your tastes. You will probably confirm that it can be difficult finding some herbs, but it is worth the effort! Also, give yourself a challenge by raising these herbs in a small garden; a 10X15 foot garden area should suffice!

Some delightful variations to use the herbs are to sprinkle them on foods and cereals. If you have a garden, as I have suggested, the greens make a delightful sandwich! Experiment and have fun constructing your sandwiches! Try other juices like apple, and tomato juice. For those who prefer you can buy the herbs in capsule form. Remember to keep this in balance with your super foods.

Below you will find information on the values of some of these key herbs. You will see how truly remarkable they are as antioxidant, circulatory, and digestive system cleaners. Hopefully, you will be impressed how valuable they are for our cellular health, tissues, skin, muscles, and bones. And, now we know of ways to bring super charged nutrients that our lives can address in DNA for our cellular life.

It is also important to realize how important chlorophyll is in our bodies. In this drink we get chlorophyll. Dangerous bacteria become weak in chlorophyll; they do not thrive in its presence. It helps cure deep lying infections, wounds, chronic sinus, and head colds. Chlorophyll helps in healing brain ulcers and pyorrhea. These herbs may prepare and have prepared the way for curing other major diseases as hepatitis, cirrhosis of the liver, etc.

HERBAL REVIEW

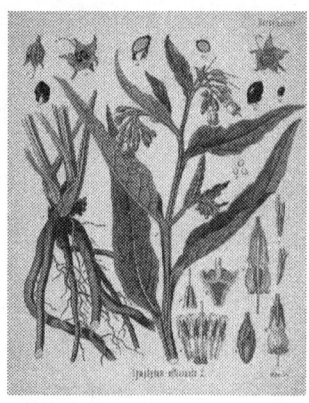

Comfrey is a gold star performer. This herb is a guardrail to prevention of diseases, including cancer. Just take care it is a variety consistent with concerns from our federal government. It can be applied directly to open wounds. Wounds will heal faster and without infection. It can be prepared as poultices. Comfrey is terrific to treat early stages of cancer, ulcers, asthma, eczema, other skin troubles, digestive disorders, boils, and varicose veins. It helps build strong bones and, yes, it aids in repair of broken bones. This herb can relieve arthritis. It is great for tuberculosis, ulcers in the lungs, alimentary canal, kidney, and gangrenous tissue problems. This is a superb herb for our health and prevention of illness.

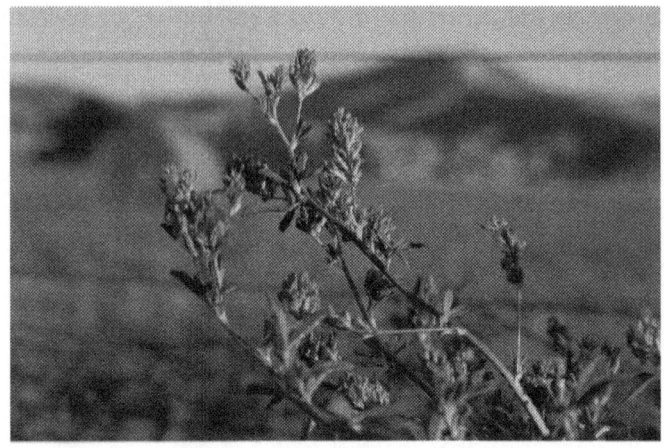

Alfalfa is dynamic in digestion and stimulates our appetite. It gives us chlorophyll too! It provides much more. Alfalfa provides enzymes, minerals, and vitamins. Alfalfa helps in digestion of the four classes of foods: protein, fats, starches, and sugars. It contains vitamin U - without this vitamin we are susceptible to peptic ulcers. It is a diuretic, helps with constipation, and other irregularities in the bowel. Alfalfa is great for bones and teeth development. It is good for those who abuse alcohol and narcotics. This herb helps with good functioning of the prostrate gland and assists recovery of many common illnesses. Alfalfa has enzymes including lipase that splits fat, has amylase that acts on starches, canales is essential for clotting of blood invertase which converts sugar to dextrose; peroxidase that helps digestion of proteins, and others. This herb is good for lumbago! Alfalfa is great for new mother's who are breast feeding their infants - think about it - cows make milk, what do they eat! Besides the vitamins of A, B, C, D, E, G, K, and U - alfalfa has amino acids: arginine, lysine, theroine, and triptophanel. This important herb also has important minerals as calcium, magnesium, sulfur, chlorine, silicon, aluminum, sodium and potassium. We should also know this herb has 150% more protein than other grains: 13.1% more protein than eggs, and 16.5% more protein than beef! It heals us, sweetens our breath, has a mild peristaltic action in the bowel, builds teeth, and stops tooth decay. Alfalfa is a fantastic grain and herb. This is a great plus in the green drink plus!

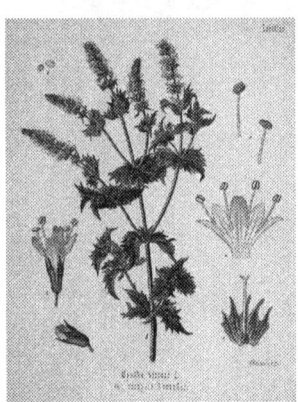

Mint flavors and makes this drink highly nutritious. It helps the body resisting and recovering from illnesses. Mint is quite soothing to our nervous system.

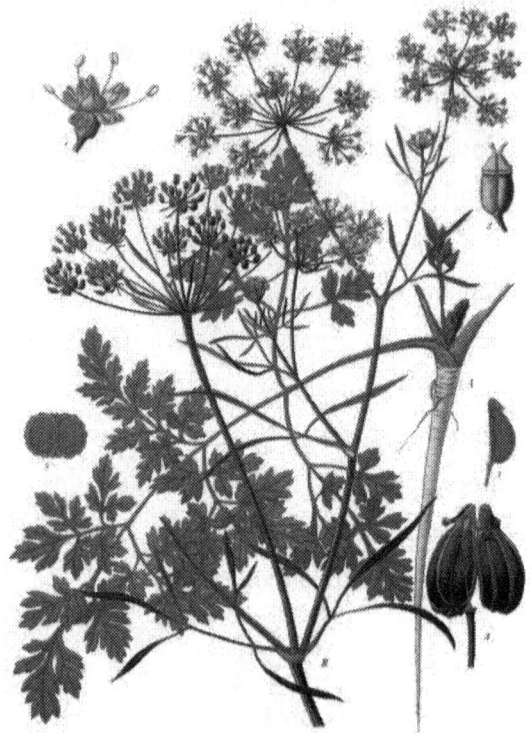

Petroselinum crispum (Mill.) Nyman ex A. W. Hill

Parsley is a great diuretic. It is excellent for genitourinary tract infections, calculi of the kidneys, bladder albuminuria, nephritis, and other kidney troubles.

Parsley helps in oxygenating our blood. It helps the normal action of the adrenal and thyroid glands. Parsley assists in preventing gallstones and eyesores.

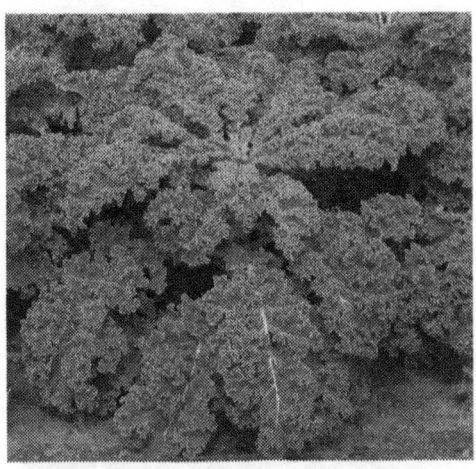

Kale or yellow dock is a laxative, a mild astringent. It purifies our blood. This herb helps us have healthy skin where scrofula and eruptions occur.

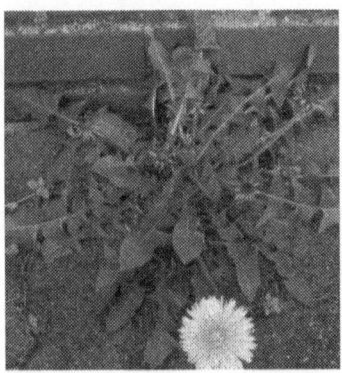

Dandelion is a mild tonic and laxative. This fine herb is good for kidney and liver disorders. It is good for those with diabetic issues. Dandelion also purifies our blood. This herb destroys acid in our blood that can cause anemic conditions.

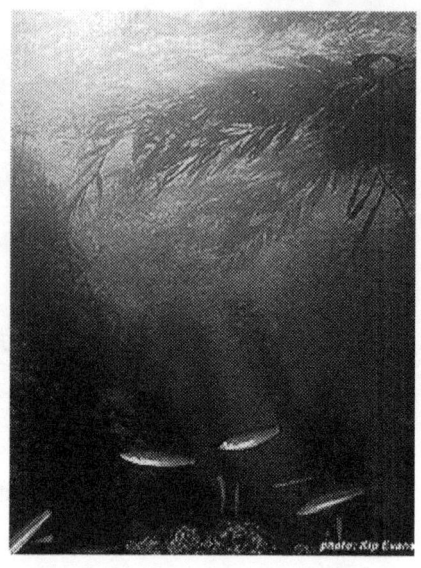

Kelp has life giving elements. It contains iodine for our thyroid gland; it has medicinal values - or healing properties. Kelp is good for our nervous system and helps our brain function normally. It has potassium, which helps treat blood pollution and prevents forms of cancer. It is a diuretic and stimulates our kidneys. Kelp helps eliminate excess water in our bodies. It helps relieve glandular diseases: goiter, rickets, anemia, and under weight issues. This herb is good for kidney disorders, eczema, neuritis, asthma, and low vitality. There are many trace minerals and elements in kelp that we need. This herb is great for our reproductive organs as prostrate, uterus, ovaries, and testes. Kelp is also good for our sensory nerves, liver, gall bladder, pancreas, bile ducts, and kidneys. It helps our large intestine clean from toxins. It helps our blood clean our arteries and restores elasticity. Kelp has nitrogen for building and repairing our body. Kelp is a big plus in this green drink!

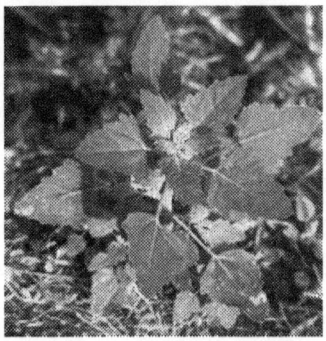

Lambs Quarter or birthroot is an astringent, antiseptic, diaphoretic, expectorant. This is good for common coughs, bronchial problems, and hemorrhages from our lungs, pulmonary consumption, and for female problems. Externally it is a great poultice for insect bites and stings.

This can become a great delight, hobby, and become a life altering way of life! You may want to add to your library some references at the end of my book. Hopefully will find a fascinating world in herbs and wonderful healthful longevity with super foods!

I invite you to begin this herbal, vitamin/super food program for a lifetime. This can become life changing, a new paradigm for living a vigorous healthy life. You will sense and know the difference within the first day, week, month, and in the years ahead. Give this at least six months to judge for yourself! You will probably have fewer colds or none to speak of; if you catch a cold you will find recovering much quicker. You may find stretching exercises will bring fewer aches and pains! Your hair will stop falling out! You will have fewer grays in your hair! Your skin around your face for example will become more youthful to half your age! Your gains will be many - please keep your own record. Remember, you can better your outcome with late developments in nutritional supplements and through the super foods. Share with your friends, family, and write Dr J your progress/story at his e-mail address: kuennenRE@aol.com. Many of us may have afflictions from our heredity. These steps will help and may, in fact, resolve them. In any case these steps are recommended to precede and/or accompany other choices. Please make sure if you are under a doctor's care, that he would be in agreement with your choice. Always check with your Doctor first. You may have some sensitivity that he may want to caution you about. I invite you to look at alternative solutions if you are dissatisfied. Otherwise, if you just want more energy. The green drink will be just for you. If you want to extend this life altering experience you will need to bring super foods into your life and learn what super charged living is about!

Should you have greater health concerns then natural solutions can bring, the next choice of what to do is very important! Check with your Alternative Medical Doctor.

To better understand your choice, see chapter 4!

CHAPTER 4

Natural Solutions or Medical Interventions:

Knowing Which to Choose!

I would like to ask you a personal question: do you believe you have a right to treat yourself? If you have a serious illness, then, when should you consult a medical professional and of what kind? Should you go to an allopathic doctor, a naturopath, a homeopath, or an alternative medical practitioner first, and why? Generally, in the United States our health care is established through the American Medical Association (AMA), allopathic medicine, who largely influence and dominate licensure of medicine in most States in the United States. Most health care providers and medical insurance companies are vested with AMA guidelines. More recently, some, insurance companies are paying alternative care providers in a few states. This makes choosing a Doctor and your future health care a bit more difficult. Who wants to pay out of their pocket when deductions for health care may already be made through their employer? What do you do when your choices may be limited, as may be the case in many locations, state and countries? Hopefully, time will help bring about a system that will be open and will continue to allow your choice of a Doctor and your choice of the kind of medicine for your medical health care. The future choices and pressures in medicine will be the determining factors in true open market systems. If your medical care system(s) are not yet fully open then you may want to become involved and alert to ways to bring this issue out.

Everyone should be alert to exercising his or her right to having a free choice in health care. Real life outcomes may be the critical difference and often are. One choice for becoming more aware and better informed is the Internet. The Internet and the news media are both providing more awareness every day! More mainstream doctors are also speaking out.

The issue of free choice may create some real challenges. If you live in a state where licensing limits choice, what do you do if your doctor insists his medicine is the only treatment for you? Or, most of us have free choice, but practically speaking if the choice is not licensable or not covered by health care systems, then what? What do most people do? The amount of one's income frames or locks in one's decision. If the knowledge and information are not openly available what should one do? Why would your Doctor not insist the best knowledge and care for your best outcome? His number one goal, even if it means exploring other medicines ought to be your best outcome? In the world there are other forms of established medicine. Allopathic medicine is the medicine most often used in the United States. Often licensure controls the only viable choice for most Americans. Who determines who can practice which medicine?

There are alternative forms of medicine that have been practiced much earlier in the history of man. There is ayurvedic medicine, recorded as early as 3,500 to 4,000 years to the Vedic civilization of India! There is the method of care through Naturopathy, a system of care handed through the generations and often identified by nutritional medical practices from treatment through colors to the use of food enrichments. There is the specialty in herbs or herbology. There are other forms of health care as well. Homeopathic's is significant for its curative goal of pathological treatment where the medicine is known. Homeopathy originally connects with Hippocrate's, view that like cures likes (similia similibus curantur). The basis of this medicine is of a "vital" rather than a physiological one. Homeopathic medicines stimulate the vital energy of a person so that he or she can be truly cured. Homeopaths believe any other drug therapy is palliative or suppressive. Other forms of treatment vary from magnetic therapy, acupressure, acupuncture, and spiritual healings or miracles. So now we can approach the notion of "Holistic medicine". This is the view that physicians don't just treat the symptoms but look for the cause of the problem, the mind, body, and spirit of a person, the totality of a person, then remove the debilitating/life threatening cause. Knowing which special form of medicine or treatment to seek is important and may be critical to continued life. This knowledge, a way to know, is one of the purposes of this book.

When we have done all we can to care for ourselves, then what? *Then…. Look for the least invasive and most curative medicine. Turning to medicine as the correct step should be considered when naturopathic ways are not effective and of course with consultation by a trusted professional.* There are situations where time is critical and a more rapid decision is required. Having a trusted holistic professional on board can be paramount. Some persons are fortunate and survive the most terminal situations, and with new knowledge many more of us should expect to do the same. Medicine as we generally know it in our western traditional form is a relatively young science. It is my belief having open medical systems that give the broadest approach for cure will allow many more persons to survive. Professional nearsightedness is not so uncommon and can be attested to daily in our many forms of media.

In 1996 I met a young man through my daughter. Both were attending a well-known State University in California. Through her, he made contact with me. He shared one of the most desperate life situations, ever, for himself. This young man drove three hours one-way to see me. He was under a traditional MD's care and one of the best specialist's care for his situation. He was no longer able to concentrate, had dropped out of college, had a girlfriend he wanted to marry but would not because of his medical condition. He reported they gave him one chance to live - to begin 18 months of interferon treatments, one shot once each month. Should he survive those treatments he was told he had a 35% chance as a recipient for a liver transplant. He reported he was diagnosed with an advanced case of hepatitis C and extensive cirrhosis of the liver. This young man believed he got this condition by helping care for a friend who had this condition. This young man did not have $1,000.00 a month for the 18 months of treatment each or $18,000.00, nor did this young man have medical coverage for a liver transplant, or for hospital care, nor for surgery expenses. I took his case information over the first two hours of his arrival. We discussed holistic care and the search for a curative medicine, which would take upwards of 25 hours of research time. We examined his life on a 24-hour times 7 days a week. We identified several things he would need to quit. He had to quit coffee that cancels some medicinal value. He had to give up all sweets, too! He left our home with a green drink plus formula while I began the research. He was to return the next weekend.

This allowed me time to do the necessary research, in order to find that one best medicine for *cure*. When he returned he had already expressed feeling better from the green drink plus. In his case his symptoms matched very well to that of a a moss prepared in homeopathic form. This was to be matched with adequate strength. Again, he left with medicine for one month. He returned feeling better but noticed loss of body heat. This required a slight adjustment in his medicine. This young man had tried many other ways including seeking a spiritual healing from God. He knew he had to get well so he could marry his sweetheart, but if he could not get well, then what? This young man was given enough medicine for one year and was to stay in touch weekly with his progress. However, he disappeared. One year later I saw him looking very well at my daughter's home during one of our visits with her at her University. This young man had returned to college with a light curriculum. He announced his intention to marry his girlfriend. He expressed his gratitude and felt the medicine derived from the moss led to his healthy return. He explained he went through tests with his past Dr and Specialist. They could not believe his recovery. What did he mean, I asked. He explained before he left, disappearing, that he was told he had no chance to survive with his case of cirrhosis and hepatitis having gotten worse and that he would not be eligible for a liver transplant had he survived the interferon treatments. The next year he had married, the following year they had a baby. It is now some seven years later and another baby in the meantime! As far as I know all are continuing in good health. Of course, this young man finished his four years of college. We thanked God together for his generosity and for the wonderful homeopathic medicines discovered by Dr Hahnemann who always gave thanks to God for his cures and discoveries of new medicines in homeopathics. If you or someone you know who wishes to consult with Dr Jay you can reach him at his e-mail: kuennenRE@aol.com.

Mixing medicines of different kinds, allopathic, homeopathic, ayurvedic is not recommended. Prevention is the first order of business. Stay healthy looking for naturopathic solutions. Be wise. Always become better informed. Do not accept limited answers - insist on openness in medicine. Help medicine to grow. Let Dr Jay know your thoughts.

The next step is to stay or become well grounded spiritually.

And, then, explore homeopathic solutions, if none are found:

Next, look to alternative medical solutions.

Finally, if no other solutions are at hand, explore traditional medicine.

It is our challenge to live wisely, fully, and until it is *His* time for us to leave this life then, hopefully receive *His* invitation in our next life. I will have more on meeting the challenge to understand in Chapter 5.

CHAPTER 5

Reaching Your Full Potential NOW –

Empowered Living to 140 and Beyond!

It is my greatest desire this brief treatise will assist all of us to reach age 140 and beyond, *empowered,* in *optimum health,* with maximum vital energy kicking up our heals celebrating life! The issue of the apocalypse will be what it will be. We can not control all things, right – right! Some things will always be a mystery. We have ways to be more prepared for important matters in life. Keep the faith! Find it if you do not have it. Sexual vitality may be an important part for you in the quest for a full long life. By accepting this quest you will come to know the difference from being strong and being ***empowered!***

Hopefully, you will have questions and ideas to share. Should you want additional source information or consult with Dr. Jay, then, within our humble constraints of time and knowledge, the process will continue!!

Despite AMA's stand to the contrary, often, there are known cures for individuals with forms of cancer, including lupus, through the middle stages of disease. Please do not doubt that Miracles do occur, also! For example many times AMA's basic understanding purported is that schizophrenia is progressive and non-curable. Yet, some persons with schizophrenia are cured! How can it be that traditional medicines' have not often lead to cure, but are talked of only in terms of remission? Why is it that traditional medicines will often complicate and all to often contribute toward early retirement of life? Yet for over 200 years homeopathics have helped many return to a full recovered life cured of disease. Other alternative medicines and treatments have their testimonials as well. And now with *super foods* individuals are walking again! Some are surviving Hepatitis C and advanced Cirrhosis of the liver, even when both were present.

I have a newsletter I publish. There is a 100% protection to you that you will be satisfied and happy by staying in touch. The newsletter is called "Kicking-up Our Heals at 140+". In this report some of my/our (my best friend and friends) latest, most delectable, food remedies are presented. Naturopathic, Ayurvedic, and Homeopathic ideas are to be found. Other health conditions with solutions will be shared. Periodically there are fun contests and the winners get excited. This newsletter is presently available yearly for just $24.95 U.S. Should you be unhappy after your first report within the first 30 days a complete refund will be made less any postage/handling costs. To get on board and begin receiving this monthly newsletter "Kicking-up Our Heals at 140+" send your money order or cashier's check to Dr J's e-mail address: kuennenRE@aol.com.

To my readers and my new friends, have a great day in Our Lord. Thank you for this opportunity to share! Let it be all our hope we see our great, great, great, great grandchildren and maybe their children before leaving this life through His Will! Then, if it can be let's look for each other in the next life!

Again, my e-mail: kuennenRE@aol.com.

Have a ***supra and super*** day, yours truly, *Dr Jay.*

REFERENCES

Awan, Malik. *Naturopathy.* Awan Publications, 1989.

Burnett, J. Compton, *Curability of Tumors.* B. Jain
Publishers, New Delhi, India.

Cherniske, Stephen, *The Metabolic Plan.* Ballantine
Books, by the Random House
Publishing Group, New York,
2003.

Giller, Robert, M. *Medical Makeover.* Beech Tree
Books, William Morrow, New
York, 1986.

Hahneman, Samuel. *Organon of Medicine.* B. Jain
Publishers, New Delhi, India.
6th Edition. 1992.

Jones, Eli G. *CANCER, Its Causes, Symptoms &*
Treatment. B. Jain Publishers,
New Delhi, India. 1991.

Kenyon, Keith. *Acupressure Cure for Common Diseases.*
Arco Publishing, Inc., 215 Park
Ave., South, New York, N.Y.
10003. 1974.

Khurana, Pushpa. *AIDS Humanity's Gravest Challenge.*
Hind Pocket Books, New Delhi,
India - 110001. 1989.

Kirschner, H.E. *Nature's Healing Grasses.* H.C. White
Publications, P.O. Box 8014, La
Sierra, California. 1962.

Laux, Marcus. *Good Health Through Age 120.* Potomac,
MD 20854. 1995.

Lust, John. *The Herb Book.* Bantam Books. New York.
1974.

Phan, Tam. *Natural Preventive Medicine.* Carlton Press,
Inc. New York, 1992.

The Record, Sat. 9-13-97, pg. 2., Stockton, California.

Santwani, M.T. *The Art of Magnetic Healing.* B. Jain
Publishers, New Delhi, India
1994.

Sastry, G.S.R. *AIDS & Homeopathy.* Curentur Homo
Publishers, Hyderabad, India.
1990.

Stout, Harry N. The Annuity Store Gazette, Vol
2, Number 2, Number 9,
September 1997.

The American Medical Association. *New Family
Medical Guide.* Random House
Publishers, Inc., New York.
1994.

University of California, Berkeley, *Wellness Made Easy.* School of Public Health, University of California, Berkeley, California. 1990.

Wallach, Joel D. BS, DVM, ND. *Dead Dr's Don't Lie.* Tape from Talk given in Kansas City, Mo. 1995 Author: Nobel Prize Nominee in Medicine. 1991.

Warrier, G. & Gunawant, D. M.D. *Ayurveda - The Ancient Indian Healing Tradition.* Element Books Inc. 1997.

Wright-Hubbard, E. Dr. M.D. *Homeopathty - A Brief Study Course.* Formur, Inc., St. Louis, Mo. 63108.

Yasgur, Jay. *A Dictionary of Homeopathic Medical Terminology.* Van Hoy Publishers, Greenville, Pa. 16125, 2nd edition. 1992.

ABOUT THE AUTHOR...

Dr Jay B. Kuennen has worked mostly in public service and has retired after 33 years of service. Twenty-seven years were in Mental Health services and six years were in Probation services, all with-in the State of California.

Jay graduated from a small high school at New Hampton, Iowa in 1960. His father was a dentist and his mother grew up on a farm. He was born at his parent's home in Garnavillo, Iowa and went to a parochial school through the third grade. Back then Garnavillo had a population of about 750. This small community is located about 5 miles from the great Mississippi river and is located in northeast Iowa. His father went into the Army and he practiced his dentistry in the Military. His father's first assignment was at Fort Leonard Wood, Missouri. Jay finished his junior high schooling in Waynesville, Missouri during those years. He attended his freshman and sophomore years of high school at Frankfurt American High School. His father was stationed in Germany during those years. On his families return to the states his father returned to private practice in New Hampton, Iowa. Dr Jay completed his junior and senior years of high school in 1960 at New Hampton High School.

After graduating from High School Jay elected to meet his military obligation and he went into the United States Air Force. He completed this obligation by serving in Turkey, Germany and Texas. He ventured to California from Iowa seeking and finding employment in State Mental Health at San Bernardino, California. While completing his Psychiatric Technician training he continued his college course work. Dr Jay completed his Associate Arts degree and his Bachelor of Arts degrees in 1968. He completed his first master's degree in Public Administration from Cal-State College, then and now is known as Cal-State University at Hayward, California in 1973. After he completed his BA degree he married in September 1968. Jay took a career move from Mental Health to corrections. He and his wife moved to Yreka, California and he took employment in Siskiyou County Probation. Their first child, a beautiful daughter was born. They moved to Martinez where he continued his Probation Officer duties.

This move was prompted out of a desire to complete his master's in Public Administration while keeping his employment with Contra Costa County. They had a second child born in 1973, another beautiful and wonderful daughter during his three years with Contra Costa County. For career opportunities they moved to Placerville, California and he went to work with El Dorado County Probation.

With a desire to raise his family in Iowa Jay and his family moved to Waterloo, Iowa. They looked forward to living closer to his aunts, uncles, and cousins. Their third child, a handsome son, was born during this time. He became the first Director of a para-legal program designed to bring equity in their criminal justice system troubled with disparities in outcome for disadvantaged persons in Blackhawk County, Iowa.

A strong sense developed for his family to return to California. Dr Jay and his wife weathered a two -year separation and divorce after returning to California. Dramatic circumstances and time brought them back together. They remarried and their fourth child, another beautiful daughter was born in Castro Valley, California. Dr Jay had formed a corporation in those years in construction. He designed and developed this corporation primarily in the energy business in the insulation and remodeling trades. They raised their children in Manteca, California. When the State's weatherization program ended Jay returned to public service in San Joaquin County Mental Health. He completed his second master's degree in Social Work before retiring on April 1, 2006. Jay had now completed about 33 years of public service.

During his years of service he accomplished service on community action committees. He continued to broaden his experiences by completing requirements for his Medical Doctorate in Homeopathics and two years later his Medical Doctorate in Alternative Medicine in 1994. By then he had acquired five State licenses from California and three Federal Security licenses. He has kept some of these licenses active including his Broker's in Real Estate license.

Doctor Jay's first marriage ended after 31 years in 1999. He now has four wonderful, responsible, and lovely children. He has four beautiful grandchildren with a fifth grandchild to be. A life person and he have found each other. She is a gorgeous, brown eyed, brunette. They are busily pursuing their lives through 140 plus years – according to God's Will, wherever their talents take them!